S. Hrg. 107–874

STATUS OF THE IMPLEMENTATION OF THE FEDERAL STEM CELL RESEARCH POLICY

HEARING

BEFORE A

SUBCOMMITTEE OF THE COMMITTEE ON APPROPRIATIONS UNITED STATES SENATE

ONE HUNDRED SEVENTH CONGRESS

SECOND SESSION

SPECIAL HEARING

SEPTEMBER 25, 2002—WASHINGTON, DC

Printed for the use of the Committee on Appropriations

Available via the World Wide Web: http://www.access.gpo.gov/congress/senate

U.S. GOVERNMENT PRINTING OFFICE

85–408 PDF   WASHINGTON : 2003

COMMITTEE ON APPROPRIATIONS

ROBERT C. BYRD, West Virginia, *Chairman*

DANIEL K. INOUYE, Hawaii
ERNEST F. HOLLINGS, South Carolina
PATRICK J. LEAHY, Vermont
TOM HARKIN, Iowa
BARBARA A. MIKULSKI, Maryland
HARRY REID, Nevada
HERB KOHL, Wisconsin
PATTY MURRAY, Washington
BYRON L. DORGAN, North Dakota
DIANNE FEINSTEIN, California
RICHARD J. DURBIN, Illinois
TIM JOHNSON, South Dakota
MARY L. LANDRIEU, Louisiana
JACK REED, Rhode Island

TED STEVENS, Alaska
THAD COCHRAN, Mississippi
ARLEN SPECTER, Pennsylvania
PETE V. DOMENICI, New Mexico
CHRISTOPHER S. BOND, Missouri
MITCH McCONNELL, Kentucky
CONRAD BURNS, Montana
RICHARD C. SHELBY, Alabama
JUDD GREGG, New Hampshire
ROBERT F. BENNETT, Utah
BEN NIGHTHORSE CAMPBELL, Colorado
LARRY CRAIG, Idaho
KAY BAILEY HUTCHISON, Texas
MIKE DeWINE, Ohio

TERRENCE E. SAUVAIN, *Staff Director*
CHARLES KIEFFER, *Deputy Staff Director*
STEVEN J. CORTESE, *Minority Staff Director*
LISA SUTHERLAND, *Minority Deputy Staff Director*

SUBCOMMITTEE ON DEPARTMENTS OF LABOR, HEALTH AND HUMAN SERVICES, AND EDUCATION, AND RELATED AGENCIES

TOM HARKIN, Iowa, *Chairman*

ERNEST F. HOLLINGS, South Carolina
DANIEL K. INOUYE, Hawaii
HARRY REID, Nevada
HERB KOHL, Wisconsin
PATTY MURRAY, Washington
MARY L. LANDRIEU, Louisiana
ROBERT C. BYRD, West Virginia

ARLEN SPECTER, Pennsylvania
THAD COCHRAN, Mississippi
JUDD GREGG, New Hampshire
LARRY CRAIG, Idaho
KAY BAILEY HUTCHISON, Texas
TED STEVENS, Alaska
MIKE DeWINE, Ohio

Professional Staff
ELLEN MURRAY
JIM SOURWINE
MARK LAISCH
ADRIENNE HALLETT
ERIK FATEMI
BETTILOU TAYLOR *(Minority)*
MARY DIETRICH *(Minority)*
SUDIP SHRIKANT PARIKH *(Minority)*
CANDICE ROGERS *(Minority)*

Administrative Support
CAROLE GEAGLEY

CONTENTS

STATUS OF THE IMPLEMENTATION OF THE FEDERAL STEM CELL RESEARCH POLICY

WEDNESDAY, SEPTEMBER 25, 2002

U.S. SENATE,
SUBCOMMITTEE ON LABOR, HEALTH AND HUMAN
SERVICES, AND EDUCATION, AND RELATED AGENCIES,
COMMITTEE ON APPROPRIATIONS,
Washington, DC.

The subcommittee met at 9:30 a.m., in room SD–124, Dirksen Senate Office Building, Hon. Arlen Specter presiding.

Present: Senators Murray, Specter, and Hutchison.

OPENING STATEMENT OF SENATOR ARLEN SPECTER

Senator SPECTER. Good morning, ladies and gentlemen. The hour of 9:30 having arrived, we will proceed with the hearing of the Appropriations Subcommittee on Labor, Health and Human Services, and Education.

Our focus today is to examine the status and implementation of the President's policy on stem cell research. Shortly after stem cells came upon the scene, the subcommittee held hearings in December of 1998, and this is our 14th hearing to follow up on this very, very important field of medical research.

The unique opportunities for the use of stem cells have been recognized in a wide variety of ailments. It has been a controversial matter because the stem cells are extracted from embryos. While there are other types of stem cells, our hearings have disclosed that embryonic stem cells are the most useful, and the opposition has focused on the possibility of life being produced by the embryos. If each embryo could produce life, that would obviously be the highest calling, but we know that thousands are thrown away. So it is my view that it is obviously preferable to use these embryos to save lives as opposed to discarding them.

The President on August 9 of last year established a policy of limiting stem cells to 63 or 67 lines, or somewhere in that range, and a big issue arises as to whether that is adequate to carry on the research.

During the course of the past year, we have had considerable controversy over nuclear transplantation which some people call therapeutic cloning, which is not cloning at all. This is a matter which is surrounded by controversy, and I think we have to find our way through because at least my view from the 14 hearings we have held is that it poses an enormous opportunity to conquer disease.

That is a relatively short opening statement to set the parameters.

The majority leader has scheduled two votes at 10:30, which means that the hearing will have to be adjourned for up to 30 minutes. I am going to do my best to move through the hearing and conclude by 10:40. I will be a little late to the first vote, but I think that is preferable than to have witnesses and observers wait a half an hour. I know how busy the people are who are at the hearing as witnesses and also as observers.

STATEMENT OF ELIAS ZERHOUNI, M.D., DIRECTOR, NATIONAL INSTITUTES OF HEALTH, DEPARTMENT OF HEALTH AND HUMAN SERVICES

Senator SPECTER. Our first witness is Dr. Elias Zerhouni, Director of the National Institutes of Health. He comes to this position with a very extraordinary record. He was executive vice dean of Johns Hopkins University School of Medicine, Chair of the Russell H. Morgan Department of Radiology and Radiological Science, and Martin Donner Professor of Radiology and Professor of Biomedical Engineering. Dr. Zerhouni received his medical degree from the University of Algiers School of Medicine, and he had his residency in diagnostic radiology at Johns Hopkins. He came to this country at the age of 24 and has had a really remarkable career.

I have already had considerable contact with Dr. Zerhouni in his first 4 months on the job, and this is his first appearance before the subcommittee. We welcome you here, Dr. Zerhouni, and look forward to your testimony.

Dr. ZERHOUNI. Thank you, Senator Specter. I am really pleased to be here this morning and testify about the role of NIH in advancing the field of stem cell research. We all know that if properly harnessed, adult and embryonic stem cells have the potential to replace cells that are damaged or diseased to restore vital functions of the human body.

There are ample reasons for excitement. I personally thought this was a field that needed to grow when I was at Johns Hopkins. There is no question that there is huge potential and promise, and high expectations for the new treatments that are possible with this approach are understandable.

But we should temper these expectations by the enormous challenges that must be addressed before the research evolves into proven therapy. I think we are at a very early stage of research in embryonic stem cell research and have a great deal of basic research to conduct before we can unlock the potential of these cells and fulfill their promise.

What I would like to do, to go over my presentation, is to use some charts to my right to go over what the basic strategy for research and research development will be in stem cell research, whether adult or embryonic. We can divide that strategy into three phases. There is the early phase called the basic research phase, and then two follow-on phases called preclinical and clinical phase.

The most important aspect of the basic research phase is for us to build the scientific capability of the field by creating career development pathways, training courses. The most important resource for any new field is trained investigators who are entering the field and advancing the field. We need to establish an infrastructure with cell culture methods, cell lines, expand the cell lines, characterize the cell line. The puzzle has to come together then in terms of us being able to both prove the long-term stability of these cells. We need to characterize them fully, and we need to make sure they are genetically stable. We need to understand the basic reason why we are so excited about stem cells is that they can differentiate and specialize into different cells in the human body. We need to understand that better at the most fundamental level, how is that done, what are the methods that we need to develop to understand this at the gene level and the molecular level. We need to understand how the cell cycle of the stem cell is controlled. One of the major risks in stem cell research is that these cells, once implanted, might revert to their more undifferentiated state and could grow into tumors. We need to understand that.

Last but not least, we have to have a lot of research go on in understanding the interactions between the cell and the host and the immunology and the transplantation biology of these cells.

As we progress, other elements of research will have to come into place. And this year we have had a lot of progress made. We have shown that in fact embryonic stem cells can differentiate into nerve tissue and insulin-producing cells. Adult stem cells have been shown to also be able to differentiate. And I believe that we should continue both embryonic stem cells and adult stem cell research at the same pace as fast as we can to go through our understanding of the puzzle that will then lead us to the preclinical phase where we need to have proof of concept experiments. We need to use the technology in animal models of disease. We need to prove what cell dosing we need to use, make sure that our understanding of tumor formation is complete, assess whether or not the cell is really functioning as we want to make it function, and eventually then, once we have accumulated that body of knowledge, go to the clinical phases of research, which are typically divided into three phases: to test whether or not there is any toxicity, what is the safety of these stem cells, and what is the efficacy of these stem cells to eventually go into therapies that will serve the public.

Now, I would like to also cover with you the work that NIH has done over the past year in trying to advance the field. There are two important elements that we as enhancers of the research, as the institution at NIH that should look to implement the research agenda—there are two resources that I consider the most critical right now.

One is the availability of researchers. So what we have done is try to develop training capabilities for researchers across the Nation. We have tried to decrease the shortage of researchers with expertise in stem cell research. We have extended additional grants to people who have expertise in stem cell research but not necessarily in human stem cell research. And we will strive to make stem cell research as attractive as possible to our most talented research scientists. So we are soliciting grant applications and I will give you some of the data related to that in a minute.

One of the most important stumbling blocks is to make human stem cells more available for research. As you know, on November 7, 2001, NIH published the registry of derived stem cells that would be eligible for Federal funding. The registry consists of 14 sources across the world. The cells are in various stages of characterization and preparation for research applications. There are many steps required to develop embryonic stem cells from when they are first removed from an embryo and put into culture into an established, well-characterized embryonic stem cell line ready for distribution to the research community.

I tried to summarize this process right here on my chart on the left side to show you what is the exact process that we need to go through to make cell lines widely available for distribution. After the derivation and the placement into culture of cells from the inner cell mass, we obtain primary colonies, which takes 3 to 5 days, the first thing we have to do is expand the primary colonies, then put them into subculture wells. Now, we need to have enough expansion of these cell lines to be able to then have enough of them to be available for distribution. The success rate here is not very high. Only 10 percent of these subcultures eventually go on to establish lines that can be characterized as human embryonic stem cell lines.

There are about 30 to 60 passages then, that have to occur to expand the number of cells within each line. As the cells divide, the total number of cells available to us for research increases. But at each passage, we need to make sure that these cells have not differentiated, and we need to have biomarkers for that purpose. We need to have ways of making sure that these cells still have the total potential of embryonic stem cells. That is done 30 to 60 times, and the expansion of these cultures is essentially the basis for the distribution that eventually occurs. It takes about 6 to 9 months to get from this stage to a stage where you have expanded these subcultures successfully, you have characterized them successfully, and one bank requires about 2 billion cells. To start to distribute these cells to the general public, you need approximately 2 million cells per vial to do so.

So the process obviously takes a while, and NIH has been very aggressive at, in fact, facilitating the availability of these cell lines from the derivations that were eligible for Federal funding. During the scaling-up process, investigators need to repeatedly check that the cells maintain their abilities, and once that is done, we can go forward with the distribution.

So as a first step, Senator, toward overcoming this challenge, NIH announced five infrastructure grant awards totaling $4.3 million to five sources on the NIH registry, holding 23 of the eligible derivations. Two additional awards have passed peer review and await final approval in funding within the next few weeks. These awards will fund the expansion, the testing, the quality assurance, and the distribution of the cells through the process I just explained.

We are also working with stem cell sources to address the complex issues that might limit widespread availability of these lines, in particular intellectual property issues. In the past year, NIH has negotiated agreements with four stem cell providers to allow both our intramural researchers access to their cells and also to allow extramural researchers to have access to these cells. Under these four agreements, six intramural laboratories at NIH have received cells to pursue research, and the agreements commit the four providers with whom we have signed agreements to offer these cells under similar terms to extramural investigators.

WARF, for example, which is the source that has been the first to be able to provide cell lines has informed us that it has agreements in place with 111 researchers and has shipped cells to 74 of them. These researchers represent 61 institutions, 12 of them in foreign countries.

Another source, ES Cell International, informs us that it currently has a supply of cells that far exceeds current demand. We are still in active discussions with all sources to be able to provide additional cell lines.

We are receiving investigator-initiated research grant applications from new investigators. So far five new grants, totaling $4.2 million, have been awarded. We have issued 32 administrative supplements to existing grant awards that allow 30 researchers from 25 different institutions to incorporate research on human embryonic stem cells as part of their ongoing federally supported research. This means that currently funded laboratories are extending their work to include human embryonic stem cells, which is a way for them to develop the skills and expertise needed in this field.

Senator SPECTER. Dr. Zerhouni, I am reluctant to interrupt you, but if you could sum up now, we would appreciate it.

Dr. ZERHOUNI. I will.

I formed a stem cell task force as soon as I arrived at NIH, and the reason I did is because I felt that it was very important for NIH to promote this field as fast as we can both in terms of embryonic and adult stem cell research. I have appointed Dr. Jim Battey as head of the Stem Cell Task Force, and I am looking forward to continue, as aggressively as we can, the development of this work. Thank you.

[The statement follows:]

PREPARED STATEMENT OF DR. ELIAS ZERHOUNI

Mr. Chairman, Senator Specter, and Members of the Subcommittee, I am pleased to appear before you today to testify about the role of NIH in advancing the field of stem cell research. Properly harnessed, adult and embryonic stem cells have the potential to replace cells that are damaged or diseased to restore vital functions of the human body. They offer the promise of curing disease and ending disabilities at some point in the future. So there are ample reasons for excitement about stem cell research, and high expectations for new treatments are understandable. But such expectations should be tempered by the enormous challenges that must be addressed before the research evolves into proven therapy.

These challenges involve both human embryonic stem cell research and adult stem cell research. Human embryonic stem cells and adult stem cells have potential as future therapies. I believe that NIH should continue to fund research on both types of cells.

We are at a very early stage of embryonic stem cell research, and have a great deal of basic research to conduct before we can unlock the potential of these cells and fulfill their promise. I will describe the pathway of discovery that I believe will unfold as the research evolves from stem cell lines to cell based therapy. In the basic research phase, which is the current focus of NIH-supported activities, we first need to build the scientific capacity. As is true for any area of research, progress depends on attracting outstanding scientists to design and perform the needed studies. NIH is providing opportunities for the scientific community to develop training courses for researchers to acquire the skills needed to culture embryonic stem cells, as well as opportunities to support stem cell research career pathways. NIH has already taken major steps to accomplish this goal by supporting infrastructure awards to expand cell lines, refine culture methods, and establish improved methods to select the most desirable embryonic stem cell populations.

There have been significant scientific discoveries in the past year involving embryonic and adult stem cells. Scientists have recently shown that human embryonic stem cells can be directed to develop into cells resembling nerve cells, cardiac muscle cells and insulin producing cells. These are the cells that might someday be used to treat Parkinson's disease, heart disease and type I diabetes.

In addition to the new research opportunity provided by the availability of human embryonic stem cells, NIH continues to aggressively support research on developing the therapeutic potential of adult stem cells. Scientists have recently discovered that adult stem cells in animals may be used to repair cartilage and bone damaged by injury and disease. In addition, research published this past summer showed that adult stem cells from the bone marrow of both rodents and humans can differentiate into multiple cell types, and can grow for long periods of time in culture. Understanding the molecular signals that direct adult stem cell differentiation may lead to new strategies for harnessing the power of a person's adult stem cells to replenish specialized cells destroyed by disease or aging. But it is clear that much more research needs to be done to explore the characteristics of adult stem cells, and to develop methods of expanding different populations of adult stem cells in the laboratory. In addition, for many types of adult stem cells, more research is needed to determine techniques to expand these cells in the laboratory, a capacity that will enable both basic and clinical studies using adult stem cells. NIH continues to believe that research on both embryonic stem cells and adult stem cells must be pursued simultaneously in order to learn as much as possible about the potential of these cells to treat human disease.

These findings are important, but I continue to emphasize that we are at a very early stage. Much more basic research needs to be done. Stem cell researchers have shown that these cells have long term viability, with no evidence for genetic changes. However, human embryonic stem cells tend to be unstable and must be closely monitored to maintain them in their undifferentiated state. Much more basic research needs to be done to validate the long term stability of human embryonic stem cells, both in culture and after transplantation. Embryonic stem cells have the remarkable capacity to continue to grow indefinitely in an unspecialized state. In research involving other cell types, much has been learned about key regulators of cell division. Additional research is needed to determine how to harness the molecular systems that control this process, so that once transplanted, the specialized cells developed from embryonic stem cells do not revert back to their embryonic state and grow in an uncontrolled fashion leading to tumors or other unwelcome outcomes.

If we are able to direct stem cells to develop into a specialized cell type, research will need to be done to determine that the specialized cells function appropriately in the context of an animal model system for human disease. NIH's long term commitment to developing such animal models for diseases such as diabetes, Parkinson's disease, and spinal cord injury will be an important factor in developing this aspect of embryonic stem cell research. As we proceed, NIH will also ensure that federal funds are used to support research that has scientific merit and demonstrates outstanding opportunities.

Such basic research is only the first phase of the journey along the pathway of embryonic stem cell research. There are many pre-clinical studies, which do not involve human subjects, that need to be performed before any new therapeutic modality advances to clinical trials on real patients. These studies include tests of the long term survival and fate of transplanted cells, cell dosing studies, as well as tests of the safety, toxicity, and effectiveness of the cells in treating animal models for disease.

Trials using human subjects, the clinical research phase, will begin only after the basic and pre-clinical foundation has been laid. This foundation will minimize any chance of unpredictable harmful effects that stem cell based therapies might cause. These trials are usually phased, with the phase I trial focusing on safety, and phase II and III trials aimed at establishing optimal dose, providing additional assurance of safety, and determining efficacy. Only after these many important steps are taken will the promise of embryonic stem cells to treat disorders like diabetes, Parkinson's disease, spinal cord injury, and cardiac failure be realized.

Having provided you with a strategic vision for research using human embryonic stem cells, I want to explain to you how NIH is addressing two immediate major issues that are essential for stem cell research community to move forward:

INCREASING THE NUMBER OF STEM CELL RESEARCHERS

As is the case at the beginning of any new field of discovery, there is a shortage of researchers with expertise in stem cell research. This dearth is currently a rate-limiting step in advancing the progress of embryonic stem cell research. Simply growing embryonic stem cells to the state where they can be used for experimentation requires substantial knowledge, training and experience. NIH will strive to make stem cell research as attractive as possible to our most talented research scientists, whose creativity in developing investigator-initiated research will move the research agenda forward. NIH is soliciting grant applications to support training courses to teach investigators how best to grow stem cells into useful lines.

MAKING HUMAN STEM CELLS MORE AVAILABLE FOR RESEARCH

On November 7, NIH published a registry of derived stem cells that would be eligible for federal funding. The registry consists of 14 sources across the world. The cells are in various stages of characterization and preparation for research applications. There are many steps required to develop embryonic stem cells from when they are first removed from an embryo and put in culture into an established, well characterized embryonic stem cell line ready for distribution to the research community. After derivation, embryonic stem cells need to be expanded from a small cluster into hundreds of million of cells before they are ready for distribution. During the scaling up process, investigators need to repeatedly check that the cells maintain their ability to divide continuously and become all of the specialized cells required for research. This process of expanding a cell line requires time, resources, and expertise.

As a first step toward overcoming this challenge, NIH has announced five infrastructure grant awards, totaling $4.3 million, to five sources on the NIH Registry holding 23 of the eligible derivations. Two additional awards passed peer review and await final approval and funding within the next few weeks. These awards will fund the expansion, testing, quality assurance and distribution of cells.

We are also working with stem cell sources to address complex issues that might limit widespread availability of these eligible cells. In the past year, NIH has negotiated agreements with four stem cell providers to allow our intramural researchers access to their cells. These providers have also agreed to offer similar terms to our grantees, enabling them to obtain cells without developing their own agreements de novo. Under these four agreements, our intramural researchers are free to publish their findings and the NIH will own any inventions made in the course of its research. As a result of these agreements, six intramural laboratories have received stem cells and are pursuing research with them. The agreements commit the four providers to offering cells under similar terms to NIH's extramural investigators. In addition, the Wisconsin Alumni Research Foundation (WARF), which holds key patents on this technology, has agreed to provide a free license to non-profit researchers conducting academic research with cells from other providers. WARF has informed us that it has agreements in place with 111 researchers, and has shipped cells to 74 of them. The researchers represent 61 institutions, 12 of them in foreign countries. Another source, ESI, informs us that it currently has a supply of cells that far exceeds current demand. Meanwhile, NIH is in active discussions with other sources listed on the NIH Registry in pursuit of additional agreements.

NIH is beginning to receive investigator-initiated research grant applications from new investigators focusing on human embryonic stem cell research. So far, five new grants, totaling $4.2 million, have been awarded. Also, NIH has issued 32 administrative supplements to existing grant awards that will allow 30 researchers from 25 different institutions to rapidly incorporate research on human embryonic stem cells as part their ongoing federally-supported research. This means that currently funded laboratories are extending their work to include human embryonic stem cells, which is a way for them to develop their skills with these difficult cells and develop some preliminary data—both key steps to success in future research. All told, over 40 investigators are now funded by the NIH to work in this area.

Much progress has occurred in the past year, including new discoveries, identifying sources of stem cells, negotiating access agreements, and creating a friendly environment to attract researchers. However, these are only initial steps. To move us into the next phase, I have created a new stem cell task force at NIH, led by Dr. James Battey, the Director of the National Institute on Deafness and Other Communication Disorders. The task force will provide direction for the future in the form of recommendations for NIH-supported research initiatives. Currently, the task force is reviewing the state of the science for all stem cell research, with the goal of using NIH resources to enable the scientific community to capitalize on this new and challenging opportunity.

NIH would not be able to move forward in stem cell research, and for that matter, any other research, without the support of this Subcommittee. Thank you for your support. I look forward to working with you to advance this and all fields of biomedical research. I will be happy to answer any questions you might have.

Senator SPECTER. Thank you very much, Dr. Zerhouni. A little more time was allowed for your presentation because of the importance of what NIH is doing in setting the stage for our other witnesses.

Since there are two votes, as I had said earlier, at 10:30, we are going to proceed now—if you would keep your seat, Dr. Zerhouni—to hear from the other five panelists, and then we will proceed to questions. So if Senator Deborah Ortiz would step forward, along with Dr. Civin, Dr. Daley, Dr. Pedersen, and Dr. Schatten, we will hear your testimony.

STATEMENT OF SENATOR DEBORAH ORTIZ, SIXTH STATE DISTRICT, CALIFORNIA STATE SENATE

Senator SPECTER. Our first witness on this panel is Senator Deborah Ortiz, elected to the 6th State Senate District in California in November 1998. She is the Chair of the Health and Human Services Committee and a member of the Education, Budget, Public Employment and Retirement, and Natural Resources and Wildlife Committees. She received her undergraduate degree from the University of California at Davis and her law degree from McGeorge School of Law.

As noted earlier, if we do not conclude by 10:40, we will have about a 30-minute break for the vote. So we are going to try to proceed to conclude at that time.

Senator Harkin could not be here today. He is the chairman and I am ranking. We traded positions last year. Senator Jeffords arranged that.

But we have had a very close collaboration, and as far as the operation of this subcommittee is concerned, it does not make any difference whether Senator Harkin is the Chair or I am. We have worked that closely.

Senator Ortiz, thank you very much for coming all the way. We look forward to your testimony. This is a clock showing 5 minutes, if you could please sum up and stop by the red light.

Ms. ORTIZ. Wonderful. Thank you, Senator Specter, as well as other members of the committee. I thank you for inviting me here. I am very conscious of running a committee on time, so I am going to pull out my watch and try to adhere to the 5-minute rule as well.

Thank you for inviting me to join you today at today's hearing as you pursue the very important question and the task of examining the implementation of President Bush's stem cell research policy and the impact of that policy on the development of stem cell technologies.

Let me begin by sharing with you why California found it imperative to move forward on stem cell research. In order to do so, let me share with you my personal history.

I served as assemblywoman and was elected to the State Assembly in 1996. As I was transitioning in my newly elected position as assemblywoman, my mother had been diagnosed with ovarian cancer. I took very seriously the task of saving her life. As I did my research and as her disease progressed, I began to understand that as important as chemotherapy and treatments like chemotherapy are in the lives of millions of cancer patients and the families who take care of those individuals, I knew that the next level of cure for cancer, as well as all the other diseases that we are all absolutely committed to curing and improving the quality of life, that the real cure really resided at a very basic level in the research, and stem cell research was offering that promise.

When President Bush declared the August 2001 64-line limitation for use in access to Federal dollars, I decided that I was going to try to have California move forward, and it became even more compelling this last spring as we began to see a couple of competing measures move through Congress. The Brownback bill posed the greatest concern to California, not just in its limitations and its criminalization of science and medicine, but also in the likelihood that there would be some success in his closing the door to science and technology and preventing the delivery of that promise to all of those Americans, over 100 million, who suffer from these diseases.

We also saw Senator Feinstein's work, and I thank the members of this committee for having often a nonpartisan debate about a very important policy issue. We were hopeful that that bill would, indeed, become law and would preclude the Brownback bill from becoming law. That was not to happen.

So as we moved forward in California, I hosted two significant hearings, one in Stanford with the brightest and most brilliant of minds, and Dr. Pedersen to my right here was good enough to videotape his testimony and welcome us from England and share with us why he left the United States in order to pursue the science that we all hope to achieve in California.

Out of that hearing at Stanford, we decided to move forward and go to the Salk Institute and also have a hearing in which Hans Keirstead, who is doing some incredible research in Irvine in California, demonstrated the mice whose spinal columns had been severed in which the introduction of stem cells produced movement and function in the lower limbs of those mice. We also heard the testimony from Jerry Zucker, the father of the 14-year-old daughter with juvenile diabetes, who shared with us his hope that his daughter would be able to live to see adulthood and not spend her life on dialysis and ultimately die at a very early age.

California decided to move forward in this research. I introduced the bill that would legalize in California stem cell research with the appropriate ethical and IRB review, as well as prohibitions for sale and transfer of embryos.

When we broadened that commitment to curing cancer, we acted decisively to pursue stem cell research in California. My law that the Governor has now signed has made, for all intents and purposes, the Bush policy on stem cell research irrelevant in the State of California. California will move forward to cure cancer, as well as Alzheimer's, as well as ALS, as well as Parkinson's, juvenile diabetes, address the spinal cord injury challenges and day-to-day realities of persons who live with those injuries. And we will move forward. We hope to share those therapies and that medical science and improvement with the rest of the country.

We ask that Congress respect California's will to protect Californians and assure that that right will be protected and not preempted by any subsequent Federal law.

California is moving forward because we understand our responsibility to pursue technology that promises to cure or effectively treat over 100 million Americans. To commit the necessary resources to deliver that hope, we have an unavoidable obligation to do everything we can do to realize the potential of stem cell research.

Once again, California is moving forward. We ask you to respect that. We believe that the Bush policy is not only medically and scientifically unsound, it is simply irrelevant in the State of California.

Thank you.

Senator SPECTER. Thank you very much, Senator Ortiz.

STATEMENT OF ROGER PEDERSEN, Ph.D., DEPARTMENT OF SURGERY, CAMBRIDGE UNIVERSITY

Senator SPECTER. We turn now to Dr. Roger Pedersen, a leading stem cell researcher, who had been at the University of California in San Francisco until September of last year. At that time, Dr. Pedersen decided to relocate to the University of Cambridge where he could receive government funding for his research on human embryonic stem cells. Currently Dr. Pedersen's research is supported by the United Kingdom Medical Research Council and the Wellcome Trust. He received his Ph.D. in biology from Yale.

We very much appreciate your coming such a long distance to join us to add your own views and insights. The necessity for your moving out of the United States is a matter of grave concern and is obviously a factor in determining what our policy should be as to stem cells. Dr. Pedersen, the floor is yours.

Dr. PEDERSEN. Senator Specter, thank you very much for the opportunity to speak.

As you know, until this time last year, I worked at the University of California, San Francisco, where I had been a faculty member for the previous 30 years and where we derived two of the novel embryonic stem cell lines on the NIH registry early last year. I now live and work in the United Kingdom where I am engaged in stem cell research at the University of Cambridge. In addition to having responsibilities for my own research team in the Department of Surgery there, I lead a consortium of 25 researchers who are focusing their individual groups on various aspects of stem cell biology and medicine. I also provide advice to other administrators and scientists in the United Kingdom who are guiding the development of the UK stem cell enterprise.

I would like to add my enthusiasm for how exciting this is as the time for stem cell researchers. We are building on more than 20 years of experience using mouse embryonic stem cells for genetic studies and on even greater experience using human blood stem cells for clinical treatments. This has provided a foundation for the successful culturing of human embryonic stem cells and opened the opportunity to control the development of human cells in the laboratory into forming a variety of useful tissues.

Importantly, we now have evidence that Dr. Zerhouni has mentioned from NIH researchers that mouse embryonic stem cells can be cultivated to produce insulin in mice and to alleviate, in other studies, the symptoms of Parkinson's in rats. These advances in stem cell biology raise our expectation for clinical benefits from stem cell medicine.

All of us know of a courageous person like Christopher Reeve who could benefit from such novel therapies. For me, it was my mother who died of diabetes in 1989, yet still provides me with an enduring will to help people with that disease. How can we achieve the clinical promise of stem cell research on their behalf?

Against these expectations, the pace of discovery of human embryonic stem cells seems painfully slow. The lack of any Federal support for research on human embryos, stretching all the way from 1978 to the present day, has undoubtedly delayed the benefits of research to infertile patients. And the long wait for Federal funding to support stem cell research has, I think, equally delayed the benefit of research to patients with degenerative diseases. I admit to having been frustrated myself with the length of time we had to wait for Federal funds for stem cell research. Admittedly, the establishment last summer of an NIH registry of human embryonic stem cells eligible for Federal funding was a significant first step in advancing such research.

However, given the length of time required to build a successful research program, any concern on the part of researchers for a worsening in the present U.S. policy for stem cell funding would tend to keep prospective researchers on the sidelines. Such concerns would definitely undermine efforts to recruit additional researchers, particularly junior investigators, into the field. It would be particularly devastating if the U.S. Senate moved to criminalize the use of somatic cell nuclear transfer to generate immune-matched stem cells. And in this respect, it is very good to see my home State of California has made clear its position in support of this and all other aspects of stem cell research.

How could the Federal Government do a better job of supporting stem cell research?

First, let me offer my respect for the will and perseverance that the NIH has shown during the last decade in their desire to support the fields of human embryology and embryonic stem cells. I believe that their approach of building up the research infrastructure by supporting training of researchers and the standardization, characterization, and distribution of the human embryonic stem cell lines on the registry will prove to be a wise one for this country. I am not convinced that it is necessary to convert the present decentralized stem cell bank to a centralized repository. Rather, I think that such a move by the NIH would lead to additional delays in the accessibility of cell lines. Therefore, my advice to them is to hold their present course.

But the truth is that the Federal Government as a whole must make a far larger commitment in order to realize the larger promise of stem cell medicine. New embryonic stem cell lines must be derived and characterized in order to meet current tissue standards for transplantation. Extensive studies are needed to define the conditions for generating large numbers of stem cell types from stem cell lines. Preclinical studies in animals, including not only rodents but also non-human primates, will be essential. And finally, careful clinical trials in appropriate patient populations will be needed to prove the efficacy of stem cells as medicines. This will all take some years to achieve. I do not believe that miracles that endure happen overnight.

To sum up my views, I believe what is needed is a long-term U.S. commitment to develop the public policies and to sustain the public funding that will make the stem cell dream come true. Why should we regard the ravages of disease as inevitable? If there is a war to be fought, surely it is against the presently untreatable diseases which kill thousands of people each day of the year. To mount an effective campaign against such diseases will require a coordinated international effort that harnesses the strength of each country. Any abdication on this front will likely cede the present U.S. leadership in the field of stem cells to Europe, Australia, or Asia, together with the economic benefits which will flow toward those countries that invest early and consistently in stem cell biology.

PREPARED STATEMENT

In closing, Senator, I would like to take this opportunity to thank you and Senator Harkin for your enduring support for this field, not only for stem cell biology and medicine, but also for all those who suffer from diseases. Thank you for hearing my views.

[The statement follows:]

PREPARED STATEMENT OF ROGER A. PEDERSEN

Honorable Senators Specter and Harkin, Distinguished Colleagues, and Guests: My name is Dr. Roger Arnold Pedersen. Until this time last year, I worked at the University of California, San Francisco, where I had been a faculty member for the previous 30 years, and where we derived two novel human embryonic stem cell lines early last year. I now live and work in the United Kingdom, where I am engaged in stem cell research at the University of Cambridge. In addition to having responsibilities in Cambridge for my own research team in the Department of Surgery, I lead a consortium of 25 researchers there who are focusing their individual groups on various aspects of stem cell biology and medicine. I also provide advice to other administrators and scientists in the United Kingdom who are guiding the development of the UK stem cell enterprise.

Now is an exciting time for stem cell researchers. We are building on more than 20 years of experience using mouse embryonic stem cells for genetic studies and on even greater experience using human blood stem cells for clinical treatments. This has provided a foundation for the successful culturing of human embryonic stem cells, opening the opportunity to control the development of human cells in the laboratory into a variety of useful tissues. Importantly, we now have evidence that mouse embryonic stem cells can be cultivated to produce insulin in mice, thus alleviating the symptoms of diabetes, and to form cells that alleviate Parkinson's symptoms in rats. These advances in stem cell biology raise our expectations for clinical benefits from stem cell medicine. All of us know of a courageous person, like Christopher Reeves, who could benefit from such novel therapies. For me it was my mother, who died of diabetes in 1989, yet still provides me with an enduring will to help people with that disease. How can we achieve the clinical promise of stem cell research on their behalf?

Against these expectations, the pace of discovery with human embryonic stem cells seems painfully slow. The lack of any federal support for research on human embryos—stretching all the way from 1978 to the present day—has undoubtedly delayed the benefits of research to infertile patients. The long wait for federal funding to support stem cell research has delayed the benefits of research to patients with degenerative diseases. I admit to having been frustrated myself with the length of time we had to wait for federal funds for stem cell research. Admittedly, the establishment last summer of an NIH registry of human embryonic stem cells eligible for federal funding was a significant first step in advancing stem cell research. However, given the length of time required to build a successful research program, any concern for a worsening in the present U.S. policy for stem cell funding would tend to keep prospective researchers on the sidelines. Such concerns could definitely undermine efforts to recruit additional researchers—particularly junior investigators—into the field. It would be particularly devastating if the U.S. Senate moved to criminalize the use of somatic cell nuclear transfer to generate immune-matched stem cells. In this respect, it is good see that my home State of California has made clear its position in support of this and all other aspects of stem cell research.

How could the federal government do a better job of encouraging stem cell research? First let me offer my respect for the will and perseverance that the NIH has shown during the last decade in their desire to support the fields of human embryology and embryonic stem cells. I believe that their approach to building up the research infrastructure by supporting training of researchers and the standardization, characterization and distribution of the human embryonic stem cell lines included on the stem cell registry will prove to be a wise one for this country. I am not convinced that it is necessary to convert the present "decentralized" stem cell bank to a centralized repository. Rather, I think such a move by the NIH would lead to additional delays in accessibility of cell lines. Therefore, my advice for them is to hold their present course.

But the truth is, the federal government as a whole must make a far larger commitment in order to realize the larger promise of stem cell medicine. New embryonic stem cell lines must be derived and characterized in order to meet current tissue standards for transplantation. Extensive studies are needed to define the conditions for generating large numbers of specialized cell types. Pre-clinical studies in animals, including not only rodents but also non-human primates, will be essential. Finally, careful clinical trials in appropriate patient populations will be needed to prove the efficacy of stem cells as medicines. This will all take some years to achieve. Miracles that endure don't usually happen overnight.

To sum up my views, I believe what is needed is a long-term United States commitment to development of public policies and sustenance of public funding that will make the stem cell dream come true. Why should we regard the ravages of disease as inevitable? If there is a war to be fought, surely it is against the presently untreatable diseases, which kill thousands of people each day of the year. To mount an effective campaign against such diseases will require a co-ordinated international effort that harnesses the strength of each country. Any abdication on this front will likely cede the present U.S. research leadership in the stem cell field to Europe, Australia or Asia. The economic benefits of stem cell medicine will flow towards those countries that invest early and consistently in stem cell biology.

In closing, I would like to take this opportunity to extend my deep appreciation to both of you, Senator Specter and Senator Harkin, for your enduring and unequivocal support, not only for stem cell biology and medicine but for all those who suffer from diseases. Thank you for hearing my views.

Senator SPECTER. Thank you very much, Dr. Pedersen.

Senator Murray.

OPENING STATEMENT OF SENATOR PATTY MURRAY

Senator MURRAY. Mr. Chairman, I am sorry to interrupt, and I have to get to a markup. If I could just ask Dr. Zerhouni one really critical question.

Senator SPECTER. Of course, Senator Murray. Proceed.

Senator MURRAY. I really appreciate your holding this hearing. I think many of us were very concerned about the President's decision to limit stem cell lines a year ago and are watching with interest that California has now move ahead on this and are very concerned what will happen in our States with perhaps a drain of researchers and where that will go.

But I just wanted to quickly ask Dr. Zerhouni if State funds are used for embryonic stem cell research, will researchers in California or any other States that enact laws like this receive NIH funds in the future, or will they be prohibited from receiving those funds?

Dr. ZERHOUNI. No. They can receive NIH funds if they work on the eligible cell lines that President's policy has identified as eligible for Federal funding. There will be no problem, and we have put in place the appropriate steps so that an investigator could work with Federal funding on eligible cell lines and work with State funding on other cell lines as desired, as currently is allowed. There is no change from what we have today.

Senator MURRAY. Thank you, Mr. Chairman. I have a number of other questions I would like to submit for the record.

Senator SPECTER. Of course, Senator Murray, they will be accepted for the record and responses will be made.

Dr. Pedersen, let me thank you for your good words for Senator Harkin and myself.

We had set upon a program to double NIH funding. We have moved it from $12 billion to $23 billion. This year we have in our budget $3.7 billion in addition. But there has to be a bill. So far we have not had any legislation come out of the appropriations process, and if we are to have a continuing resolution, that means that the funding will probably stay level. That will be very, very bad for many projects, but especially for NIH where we will have done more than the doubling which we had anticipated. From $12 billion, it would put us at $26.7 billion.

I make that comment at this time so that all of those here can use your lobbying influences to help us get a bill, and if you want a more particular road map, I would be glad to talk to you later.

STATEMENT OF GERALD SCHATTEN, Ph.D., PROFESSOR OF CELL BI-OLOGY, UNIVERSITY OF PITTSBURGH, DIRECTOR, PITTSBURGH DEVELOPMENT CENTER, AND DEPUTY DIRECTOR, MAGEE-WOMEN'S RESEARCH INSTITUTE

Senator SPECTER. We will turn now to Dr. Gerald Schatten, deputy director of Magee-Women's Research Institute and director of the Pittsburgh Development Center. He is a professor and vice chair of obstetrics, gynecology and reproductive sciences and cell biology at the University of Pittsburgh School of Medicine. He received his Ph.D. from the University of California at Berkeley.

I have worked with you and, we are glad to have you in Pennsylvania, Dr. Schatten. It seems to me we have got a very heavy California influence here today.

The floor is yours.

Dr. SCHATTEN. Thank you, Senator Specter, and it is a great pleasure for me to have this opportunity to speak with you.

The NIH deserves tremendous commendations for their efforts in rapid implementation this past year, but serious and substantial work remains. From my own experiences, I need to voice grave concerns about the current Federal stem cell policies because it is already hindering invaluable research, undermining the wisest investments, and delaying the day when we will know for sure whether human embryonic stem cells can be used to treat diseases.

The NIH's registry lists 71 lines. Science reports only 16 are available. My search has identified just a handful. As of last Thursday, we have just two.

We need accuracy and clarity. Perhaps 71 lines do meet eligibility criteria, but just being eligible is not the same as available.

To obtain approved lines, I have traveled to Europe and Asia to collaborate with scientists in Korea, Singapore, Australia, Sweden, and the UK. They are willing and motivated. But should American science not also be conducted on American soil?

NIH has sponsored my research for the last 25 years, and we investigate how fertilization succeeds and how the embryo develops. Last November, we were among the first to apply to investigate how human embryonic stem cells divide and proliferate. When cells lose chromosomes, they can develop into cancers. If human embryonic stem cells lose chromosomes when they are put into a patient's body, as Dr. Zerhouni mentioned, they could develop into cancers. Chromosome movements in human embryonic stem cells must be accurate and that is just what we are doing in our laboratory.

Researchers at the Pittsburgh Development Center of Magee-Women's are discovering that embryos form very differently between the mammals cloned successfully by somatic cell nuclear transfer and primates, as investigated in monkeys. Cloned cows and mice can develop without any sperm contributions, whereas primates, in which all somatic cell cloning attempts have failed so far, appear to depend on a unique complementation between the egg's machinery and the sperm's special structures.

Reproductive cloning in humans is dangerous, unethical, unjustified, and for biological purposes we would predict that it will fail.

Therapeutic cloning, on the other hand, in which embryonic stem cells are produced in a plastic dish in the absence of any sperm or any fertilization event, promises unique methods to overcome our body's own immune rejection systems. The editorial this week in Science entitled "Harmful Moratorium on Stem Cell Research" is authored by some of the hand-picked members of the President's own Bioethics Panel.

Last April, NIH modestly funded our proposal for just a year. These supplements are insufficient in time or amount for the best research programs to justify redirection. The NIH must be more aggressive in supplementing investigator-initiated grants with significant funding. Cooperative agreements would enlarge the talent pool. New equipment is necessary to ensure the separate of stem cell research from ongoing activities. Labs selected for multi-year awards should also be responsible for research training.

Commercial-academic cooperations also need to be encouraged further.

On Sunday, I met with Lans Taylor, who is CEO of the Pittsburgh-based company Cellomics. He has mocked up human embryonic stem cell pluripotency kits and assays to determine whether these lines will develop into neurons. Other companies could further reduce the hurdles very swiftly if they were encouraged to jump into this field and reduce the research hurdles.

During this hearing, we have discussed national policy and contrasted it with stem cell rules elsewhere. We are the United States and each State has its own laws and restrictions that may prove enabling or restrictive. Senator Specter, you know well that our Commonwealth of Pennsylvania has language restricting human embryonic stem cell research. The Abortion Control Act of 1989, written long before stem cells were discovered, prohibits embryonic research.

Homeland Security Director Tom Ridge, while still Governor of Pennsylvania, decided that cells derived outside of Pennsylvania were eligible for research within our commonwealth.

We have heard just now from Senator Ortiz that California is enacting laws to enable human embryonic stem cell studies.

It may be within this subcommittee's purview that in addition to witnessing American scientists emigrating, we may soon see U.S. scientists relocating from States with ambiguous laws to other States.

Senator Specter, subcommittee members, I applaud you and others in Congress for your unwavering support of the NIH. Your sponsorship and encouragement of healthy Federal and private sector competition produced the human genome sequence under budget and far sooner than expected. When we decided to decipher the genome, which also generated controversies, we deliberated thoughtfully and invested adequately.

More and better lines are needed now and current policies are already delaying stem cell research, forcing it off shore or into inaccessible reaches in the private sector.

PREPARED STATEMENT

Would Galileo have been satisfied if he could have looked at 65 or 71 stars? Maybe, but he would not have discovered our place in the solar system unless Jupiter traveled through that narrow field.

In today's terms, the cost of the Hubble telescope and all of NASA is the same if our focus is restricted or if we are permitted to explore the heavens.

Thank you.

[The statement follows:]

PREPARED STATEMENT OF DR. GERALD SCHATTEN

Good morning, Chairman Harkin, Senator Specter, and other distinguished Subcommittee Members. I'm Gerald Schatten, Professor of Cell Biology at the University of Pittsburgh and Director of the Pittsburgh Development Center.

The NIH deserves commendation for their efforts and rapid implementation this past year, but serious and substantial work remains. From my experiences, I need to voice grave concerns about the current federal stem cell policy because it's already hindering invaluable research, undermining the wisest expenditures and delaying the day when we'll know whether stem cells can be used to treat diseases.

The NIH's Human Embryonic Stem Cell Registry lists 71 lines. SCIENCE reports only 16 are available. My search has identified just a handful right now—as of last Thursday, we've received two.

We need accuracy and clarity. Perhaps 71 lines meet eligibility criteria, but just being eligible isn't the same as available.

To obtain approved lines, I've traveled to Europe and Asia to collaborate with scientists in Korea, Singapore, Australia, Sweden and the UK. They're willing and motivated . . . but American science should also be conducted on American soil.

NIH has sponsored my team's research for the past twenty-five years and we investigate how fertilization succeeds and how the embryo forms. Last November, we were among the first to apply to investigate how human embryonic stem cells divide and proliferate. When cells lose chromosomes, they can develop into cancers. Chromosome movements must be accurate in HESCs for safe transfer to patients, or new cancers might arise—and that's what we're working to understand and prevent.

Researchers at the Pittsburgh Development Center are discovering that embryos form very differently between the mammals cloned successfully by somatic cell nuclear transfer (SCNT) and primates, as investigated with monkeys. Cloned cows and mice can develop without any sperm contributions, whereas primates, in which all SCNT cloning attempts have failed so far, appear to depend on the unique complementation of the egg's essential machinery with special sperm's structures.

Reproductive cloning in humans is dangerous, unjustified and unethical.

Therapeutic cloning, in which embryonic stem cells are produced in a plastic dish in the absence of any sperm or fertilization event, promises unique methods to overcome our body's natural immune rejection systems. The editorial this week in SCIENCE entitled "Harmful Moratorium on Stem Cell Research" is authored by some of the handpicked members of the President's Bioethics Panel.

Last April NIH modestly funded our proposal for just one year. These supplements are insufficient in time or amount for the best research programs to justify redirection. The NIH must be more aggressive in supplementing investigator-initiated grants with significant, not token, funding. Cooperative agreements would enlarge the pool of talented labs. New equipment is necessary both to ensure the separation of HESC research from on-going lab activities and also because the tests for pluripotency and differentiation are specialized. Labs selected for multi-year awards could be responsible for research training.

Commercial-academic cooperation needs to be encouraged further. As one example, I asked Lans Taylor, CEO of Cellomics to mock up pluripotency, growth and differentiation assays. Pittsburgh-based Cellomics and other companies could further reduce research hurdles quickly.

During this hearing, we've discussed our national policy and contrasted it with stem cell rules elsewhere. We are united States—and each state has its own laws and regulations that may prove enabling or restrictive.

Senator Specter knows well that our Commonwealth of Pennsylvania has language restricting HESC research. The Abortion Control Act of 1989, written long before HESCs were discovered, prohibits embryonic research.

Homeland Security Director Tom Ridge, while still Governor of Pennsylvania, decided that cells derived outside of Pennsylvania were eligible for research within our commonwealth.

We've all read that California is enacting laws to enable HESC studies.

It is may be within this subcommittee's purview that in addition to witnessing American scientists emigrating, we may soon also see U.S. scientists relocating from States with ambiguous laws to other States.

Mr. Chairman, Senator Specter, Subcommittee Members, I applaud you and others in Congress for your unwavering support of NIH—your sponsorship and encouragement of healthy federal and private sector competition produced the human genome sequence under budget and sooner than predicted. When we decided to decipher the Genome, which also generated controversies, we deliberated thoughtfully and invested adequately.

More and better lines are needed now and current policies are already delaying stem cell research, forcing it offshore or into inaccessible reaches in the private sector.

Would Galileo have been satisfied if he could have looked at 59 or 71 stars? Maybe, but he wouldn't have discovered our place in the Solar System unless Jupiter traveled through that narrow field.

In today's terms, the cost of the Hubble telescope and all of NASA is the same if our focus is restricted, or if we're permitted to explore the heavens.

Thank you.

Senator SPECTER. Thank you, Dr. Schatten. Dr. Schatten, you are safe in Pennsylvania. Do not move.

STATEMENT OF CURT CIVIN, M.D., PROFESSOR OF CANCER RESEARCH, SIDNEY KIMMEL COMPREHENSIVE CANCER CENTER, JOHNS HOPKINS UNIVERSITY

Senator SPECTER. We turn now to Dr. Curt Civin, King Fahd Professor of Oncology at Johns Hopkins University where he developed a stem cell selection process which has led to the development of more effective and less toxic cancer therapies. Dr. Civin holds nine patents for biomedical inventions related to stem cell research. He received his M.D. from Harvard Medical School.

Thanks for joining us, Dr. Civin, and we look forward to your testimony.

Dr. CIVIN. Thank you, Senator Specter, Senator Hutchison, Senator Ortiz. Thank you for the honor of testifying before you today.

I am very grateful for this committee's strong and consistent support for lifesaving biomedical research. It is also a special privilege for me to testify today with my friend and former Johns Hopkins colleague, Elias Zerhouni. Our Nation is indeed privileged to have a scientist of his distinction and capability serve as NIH Director.

I am professor of Cancer Research at the Johns Hopkins University School of Medicine, where I hope to stay. My clinical specialty is caring for children with cancer and this motivates my research. For the past 23 years, I have studied adult stem cells, mainly human bone marrow stem cells that can reconstitute our blood and immune systems. I discovered the CD34 stem cell molecule that allows identification and isolation of these rare blood-forming stem cells. The discovery is widely used in stem cell research and in clinical bone marrow transplantation, and two companies have licensed related inventions. And so I want to disclose to you that Johns Hopkins University and I have a financial interest in certain stem cell inventions and medical therapies.

Today my research continues to focus on adult stem cells. We need to figure out how to grow these stem cells easily and in large numbers so that, for example, a bone marrow donation from one single donor can provide enough stem cells for multiple transplant patients.

The 1998 discovery of human embryonic stem cells significantly raised our hopes of solving this therapeutic problem. By studying these cells, we hope to discover the molecular pathways by which they can proliferate without differentiating and then figure out how, in effect, to push the same molecular buttons in adult stem cells. Such discoveries would enhance the treatment of my cancer patients and might also help in the development of stem cell regenerative medical therapies for the range of other diseases.

President Bush's decision to allow federally funded research on a qualified number of human ES stem cell lines increased our hopes of advancing this research. The decision has, however, proved much more limited than we anticipated. More than a year after the President's announcement, I am still waiting to receive my very first stem cell line. In fact, embryonic stem cell research is crawling like a caterpillar. Few human embryonic stem cell lines exist and most are not truly available. A number of the lines on the NIH stem cell registry have been tied up in questions of ownership. Many of the owners of the not-in-dispute cell lines are not anxious to share them with other researchers. Those that are willing to share their lines expect a piece of the profits on future discoveries. The terms of material transfer agreements are often difficult and time consuming to negotiate. The owners also expect an up-front fee. The going rate is $5,000, an amount 50 to 100 times greater than what we are accustomed to paying for a cell line.

Besides these administrative burdens, there are significant technical challenges as well. Little is known about the cell lines themselves. Without this information, individual researchers are essentially flying blind. We must characterize the cell lines ourselves, an extraordinarily inefficient use of limited resources.

An example. Last fall, a colleague applied to receive the best studied of the cell lines on the initial NIH list, the H1 cell line from Wisconsin. Six months later he received the cells. It took him more than 4 months to grow enough ES cells to perform even preliminary experiments. These cells grow exceedingly slowly, one-tenth the rate of the cells we usually work with.

For my research, I need several ES cell lines since I am sure that not all will form blood cells or will grow rapidly. Last fall I was contacted by a company in India which owns seven of the embryonic stem cell lines on the NIH registry. They wanted to collaborate with my lab to explore the blood-forming potential of these lines. I spent several months negotiating collaboration and materials transfer, but the imminent agreement was abruptly canceled in May. The company told me that the Indian Government had put an indefinite hold on sending ES cell lines out of their country.

In July I applied for a different ES cell line from Wisconsin that is reported to grow somewhat faster than H1 and to form some blood cells. I have been told that because of technical problems with these cells, I will not receive them until October at the earliest.

Stem cell research has tremendous potential to deliver treatments and cures. With research we can make stem cells that are self-renewing, that are less likely to be rejected by the recipient's immune system and that regenerate tissues and organs fully.

Today the United States of America is the best place in the world to do all biomedical research. I do not want us to lose that lead in stem cell research. And we are really in danger of doing so. Without our vigorous leadership in federally supported research in this country, the worldwide pace of discoveries will be much slower than necessary. Instead of being the first in line to benefit from new treatments as they are now, our patients in America will have to wait. We will lose talent to other nations, as you have heard, and new jobs and industries will be spawned elsewhere.

Every week we read about exciting new stem cell research underway in other countries. Prime Minister Tony Blair of the UK recently said he wants Britain to be the best place in the world for stem cell research. Singapore has invested $1.7 billion. I am heartened by Dr. Zerhouni's recent creation of the NIH Stem Cell Task Force and look forward to its contributions. Much work needs to be done.

Mr. Chairman, I am also, again, grateful to the subcommittee for including language here in your fiscal year 2003 committee report directing NIH to take positive steps to stimulate research. Specifically I would strongly endorse your language, urging NIH to develop a stem cell repository. A repository would promote research and lower the barriers to obtaining stem cell lines for investigators like me. Under this arrangement, NIH would characterize the lines and then act as a technical resource and distribution center. This would eliminate duplication of effort and provide an invaluable technical resource for growing the cells.

PREPARED STATEMENT

Once again I want to thank you for your commitment to biomedical research and for your assistance in clearing unnecessary impediments to progress. You have really made a difference. Thank you.

[The statement follows:]

PREPARED STATEMENT OF DR. CURT I. CIVIN

Chairman Harkin, Ranking Member Specter, and members of the Subcommittee thank you for the honor of testifying before you today about the hurdles that I, and many other, scientists have experienced in attempting to conduct embryonic stem cell research in the wake of President Bush's decision last year to permit research on a qualified number of stem cell lines. I am very grateful for your strong and consistent support of biomedical research and your interest in promoting life-saving stem cell research. I am also grateful for the language included in your fiscal year 2003 Committee Report directing NIH to take a number of positive steps to stimulate stem cell research.

I am Professor of Cancer Research at the Sidney Kimmel Comprehensive Cancer Center of the Johns Hopkins University School of Medicine. My clinical specialty is caring for children with cancer, and this motivates my laboratory research on normal and leukemic stem cells. For the past 23 years, I have studied adult stem cells, mainly the stem cells from human bone marrow that can reconstitute our blood and immune systems after intensive radio-chemotherapy in a bone marrow transplant. I am best known scientifically for discovery of the CD34 stem cell molecule that allows identification and isolation of these rare blood-forming stem cells. The CD34 monoclonal antibody is widely used in stem cell research as well as clinical bone marrow transplantation, and for this I received the National Inventor of the Year Award in 1999. Thousands of patients have received successful bone marrow stem cell transplants, mainly to mediate the toxic effects of their cancer therapy, but also for diseases such as immune deficiencies, autoimmune disorders, and aplastic anemia. Two companies have licensed related inventions, and so I must disclose to you that Johns Hopkins University and I have a financial interest in certain stem cell research and medical therapies.

Today, my research continues to focus on adult stem cells. Despite our successes, over 15 years of intense investigations on adult blood-forming stem cells has not taught us all we need to know about the biology of these adult stem cells. For example, we need to figure out ways to grow these cells easily and in large numbers so that like yeast in a fermenter a marrow donation from one donor could be expanded to provide stem cells for multiple bone marrow transplant recipient patients. The problem is that, outside of the body, these blood-forming stem cells rarely proliferate without differentiating. That is, the stem cells divide into more mature progeny that are no longer stem cells.

So I was excited by the 1998 discovery of human embryonic stem cells (hES) that can expand indefinitely in tissue culture without losing their capacity to generate stem cells of many types of organs and tissues. Our hope is to study these embryonic stem cells, discover the molecular pathways by which they can proliferate without differentiating, and then figure out how, in effect, to push the same molecular buttons in adult stem cells. Such discoveries would enhance the treatment of my patients with cancer, by using transplants of adult stem cells taken from bone marrow. In addition, the lessons from this research might also help in the development of stem cell regenerative medical therapies for a range of other diseases. Note that the ultimate goal of my research is to facilitate the use of adult stem cells in the clinic by studying embryonic stem cells in the laboratory.

In the years 1998–99, I was able to study a single line of human embryonic germ cells that was derived at Johns Hopkins. I had to be exceedingly careful not to use any federal funds to do these studies. Corporate agreements slowed and limited extensive experiments. Unfortunately, our research did not find the key to unlock the mechanisms that could turn this cell line into blood-forming cells. One possible reason is that this cell line seemed to have a predilection to develop into nerve, not blood cells. I then needed to obtain several other cell lines for further studies. Federal policy decisions in 2000/2001 appeared to allow me to do this. However, these guidelines were put on hold in early 2001, until President Bush announced the current guidelines in August 2001, more than a year ago.

The President's decision renewed our hopes of pursuing this therapeutic research. NIH's initial list of stem cell lines that could be used in federally funded research seemed like a straightforward source of available resources. However, we quickly found out that none of these cell lines was available readily to us. That remains true today.

In fact, embryonic stem cell research is crawling like a caterpillar. While NIH has listed more eligible lines on its registry (http://escr.nih.gov/), only a tiny fraction of these lines are accessible—and only to those persistent and patient enough to jump through a series of hoops and endure lengthy waits. I am still waiting to receive my first stem cell line.

The difficulties are numerous. As recent news articles have reported, and my experience has shown, some of the lines have been tied-up in questions of ownership. Many of the owners of lines, not in dispute, are not anxious to share them with other researchers. Those that are willing to share the lines, are not willing to do so without getting a piece of the profits of future discoveries made using the lines. The terms of material transfer agreements are often difficult and time-consuming to negotiate. The owners also expect an upfront fee. The going rate is $5,000—an amount 50–100 times greater than the $50–$100 we are accustomed to paying for a cell line.

While the administrative burdens necessary to obtain stem cells from NIH's list of eligible lines are tremendous and the costs significant, little is known about the lines themselves. Without this information, individual researchers are essentially flying blind. They must characterize the lines themselves and determine through a painful process of trial and error whether any line will advance their research. This is an extraordinarily inefficient use of limited resources.

The best studied of the cell lines on the initial NIH-approved list was the H1 cell line from Wisconsin. A colleague of mine applied to receive these cells in fall, 2001. Finally six months later, after complex material transfer negotiations and a $5,000 payment, he received the cells. Having cleared the administrative and financial hurdles, the next problem he confronted was technical. These cells grow exceedingly slowly, one-tenth the rate of the cells we usually work with. So it has taken my colleague more than four additional months of incremental steps until he has been able to grow enough ES cells to perform even preliminary experiments.

I need several ES cell lines, since I suspect from prior experience that not all will form blood cells, or grow rapidly. In Fall 2001, Reliance Life Sciences, a company from India contacted me. One of Reliance's scientists had been the Ph.D. mentor for a current postdoctoral fellow in my lab, and he knew our work well. Seven of the ES cell lines on NIH's current list of 81 approved hES cell lines are owned by Reliance, and they wanted to collaborate with my lab to explore the blood-forming potential of these cell lines. I spent several months negotiating collaboration and materials transfer, but the imminent agreement was abruptly cancelled in May 2002. The company told me that the Indian government had put an indefinite hold on sending human ES cells out of their country.

Another ES cell line from Wisconsin, called H9, is reported to grow somewhat faster than H1, and to form some blood cells. Having learned in June 2002, that H9 cells would be available in July, I applied for this cell line. I completed the now simpler material transfer forms, and paid my $5,000, but I have been told that because of some technical problems with the H9 cells, I will not receive them until October, at the earliest. I look forward to these experiments, but despair of being able, in the near future, to obtain or afford multiple ES cell lines for the research I would like to do.

My experience obtaining stem cells from NIH's approved list is not unique. This paper chase for stem cell lines has stunted the field of stem cell research. Most investigators need multiple hES cell lines. Few hES cell lines exist, and most are not truly available. In fact, it is my understanding that only the cells from Wisconsin and, as of just last week, one cell line from the University of California, San Francisco are available to scientists who are neither collaborators of the companies nor investigators who derived the lines. Only a few federal grants are trickling out for stem cell research. The review of a grant application is always rigorous. Scientist peer-reviewers demand that the applicant demonstrate experience with the cells and model systems proposed, and some strong preliminary results showing that the concepts proposed for investigation are not just wishful thinking. This has served as a Catch–22 for many scientists who want to study human ES cells, since the human ES cell lines they need simply to begin their research are few and costly, they grow very slowly, and the available cell lines may not be able to function as needed, as in my case to develop blood, or other specific tissue types.

Many scientists have similar stories to tell, and you will hear from several eminent ones today. We all believe that stem cell research has tremendous potential to deliver treatments and cures. I believe that the pressure should be on us, as stem cell researchers to turn that potential into treatments for our patients. With research, we can make stem cells that are self-renewing, that are less likely to be rejected by the recipient's immune system, and which regenerate a variety of engineered tissues and organs that might even perform better than the originals. As a scientist, I want to get started. I want to bring these benefits to my patients and others. I do not want to limp along. I want other scientists to enter this field. I want to be spurred on by their advances.

Today, the USA is the best place in the world for every field of biomedical research. I do not want us to lose that lead in stem cell research—and we are in danger of doing so. Without our vigorous leadership in federally supported stem cell research, the pace of discoveries will be much slower than necessary. Instead of being the first in line to benefit from new treatments developed at home, Americans will have to wait. We will lose talent to other nations. And, new jobs and industries will be spawned elsewhere.

Every week, we read about exciting new stem cell research underway in countries, many of which have not been known, historically, as leaders in biomedical research. The list includes China, Singapore, Australia, and the U.K. *The Financial Times* reports that Prime Minister Tony Blair wants to make Britain the "best place in the world" for stem cell research, so that "in time our scientists, together with those we are attracting from overseas, can develop new therapies to tackle brain and spinal cord repair, Alzheimer's disease, and other degenerative diseases such as Parkinson's." [1] Singapore shares these ambitions. *The Economist* reports that the Asian nation seeks to become a magnet for stem cell research. In the last two years alone, it has invested $1.7 billion in efforts to attract global talent and industry and build its infrastructure to support stem cell research. [2]

I believe it is our nation's responsibility and indeed in our interest not to let the discoveries, the treatments and cures, and the jobs that stem cell research will someday provide move overseas. We need to pursue all promising avenues of stem cell discovery. U.S. scientists need better access to human embryonic stem cells to continue to lead the field of stem cell research.

I am heartened by NIH Director Elias Zerhouni's recent creation of a Stem Cell Task Force and look forward to its contributions to the field. Much work needs to be done to reduce administrative and technical barriers and to encourage more scientists to pursue this vital research.

I also strongly endorse your fiscal year 2003 Committee Report language on stem cell research, urging NIH to develop a stem cell repository. Such an initiative would promote research by lowering the costs—in both time and money—of obtaining stem cell lines. Under this arrangement, NIH would characterize the cell lines, and then act as a technical resource and distribution center for scientists seeking to obtain them. This would eliminate duplication of effort and provide an invaluable technical resource for growing the cells. Vesting one organization with the ability to distribute all cell lines would also produce economies of scale.

Once again, Mr. Chairman and members of the subcommittee, I want to thank you for your commitment to biomedical research and for your assistance in clearing unnecessary impediments to progress.

Thank you very much, Dr. Civin.

STATEMENT OF GEORGE DALEY, M.D., Ph.D., ASSISTANT PROFESSOR OF MEDICINE, HARVARD MEDICAL SCHOOL; AND FELLOW, WHITEHEAD INSTITUTE FOR BIOMEDICAL RESEARCH

Senator SPECTER. Our next witness is Dr. George Daley, assistant professor of Medicine at Harvard and a fellow at the MIT-affiliated Whitehead Institute where he studies stem cells of the blood. His research has helped define the molecular basis for human leukemia and provided insights into normal blood development. Prior to his appointment at Harvard, Dr. Daley served as chief resident in medicine at Massachusetts General Hospital. His Ph.D. is from MIT and his M.D. is from the Harvard Medical School.

Welcome, Dr. Daley. We look forward to your testimony.

Dr. DALEY. Thank you, Chairman Specter, distinguished members of the subcommittee.

My name is George Daley. I am a faculty member at Harvard Medical School and I run a research laboratory at the MIT-affiliated Whitehead Institute that studies stem cells that the body uses to form blood. This has prompted our intense interest in using human embryonic stem cells for our research. My laboratory currently holds NIH grants to support research on both mouse and human embryonic stem cell biology.

---

[1] "The stem of competitiveness," The Financial Times, August 30, 2002.
[2] "Send in the clones," The Economist, August 24, 2002 U.S. Edition.

My laboratory has spent the last 7 years using mouse ES cells to investigate how blood cells develop in the Petri dish. Recently our group has taken a step forward. We successfully transplanted mice with blood stem cells derived entirely from mouse embryonic stem cells. Then, in collaboration with my colleague, Rudolf Jaenisch, we performed an important first demonstration of therapeutic cloning to treat a mouse with a genetic immunodeficiency, similar to the Bubble-boy disease. Our team plucked a cell from the tail of an afflicted mouse, used nuclear transfer to create an ES cell line, used gene therapy to correct the genetic defect, and then performed blood stem cell transplants into diseased mice. The repaired ES cells provided a source of immune cells and antibodies in the treated mice.

Encouraged by this first proof of principle in an animal model, my team is eager to apply the same strategy to human ES cells. Our hope is that one day the process will be efficient, safe, and effective for treating patients with a variety of genetic and malignant bone marrow diseases.

However, over the past year, the progress of my own team and I would say that of the research community in general has been palpably slowed, in part because of the frustrating lack of access to human ES cells and in part due to the restrictive nature of the President's funding policy as mandated in his address of August 9, 2001.

I wish to make three points.

First, the biomedical research community needs more cell lines. While the President announced that over 60-odd lines were available, it has become increasingly clear over the past year that far fewer lines have been characterized adequately, perhaps only a handful.

Second, the research community needs a central repository for ES cell lines, preferably in a facility funded by NIH, that would provide free access to a comprehensive set of carefully maintained and documented lines for research.

Third, I wish to emphasize that the Federal funding guidelines are currently so restrictive that they are already threatening this fledgling, yet highly promising field of research.

First, my personal experience. My team was one of the first in the United States to gain access to the ES cells that Jamie Thomson and his colleagues derived at the University of Wisconsin. However, since obtaining that single cell line in mid-2000, we have been frustrated in attempts to obtain another. One week ago, after nearly 2 years of inquiries with a number of other research groups, we finally received our second line.

Why did it take so long? Well, the number of laboratories interested in working with these cells is increasing explosively. This dictates that a more effective means must be established for the distribution of these valuable reagents. I believe that a central warehouse and processing facility should be established and funded by the NIH. A central repository would maintain consistent, standard operating procedures for the culture and maintenance of the cell lines.

Finally, I want to comment on the state of research on human embryonic stem cells after a year under the policy announced by

President Bush last August. I would applaud President Bush for his principled stance in favor of human ES cell research. Having access to even a few well-characterized human ES cell lines enables us in the research community to begin to address generic questions about ES cell biology. However, this is only the beginning and the current policy will not enable the research community to follow through with the work needed to treat patients. President Bush made the right call in allowing Federal funding for research, but his policy excludes some of the most important and promising new avenues.

As I have stated, it is unclear precisely how many cell lines exist, but I strongly believe that the number is far fewer than listed on the NIH registry.

Second, the President's policy does not allow support for deriving new cell lines which is of tremendous scientific interest.

My last point, the President's policy does not allow for studies of ES cell lines derived by nuclear transfer. This is currently the most appealing avenue for creating ES cells from patients with specific diseases and for creating ES cell lines that are genetically matched to patients. Our research team showed that nuclear transfer methods can be applied in the practice of therapeutic cloning in mice. I have no doubt that legitimate and successful medical treatments in real patients will be developed sooner if the Federal Government funds nuclear transfer studies with human ES cells starting today. The sad and undeniable truth is that the existing restrictions are keeping these advances from being realized.

PREPARED STATEMENT

In conclusion, I would say that the field of ES cell research is in a fragile state at best under the current presidential policy. The current policy represents a half-hearted effort to support this revolution in biology and threatens to starve the field at a time when greater nourishment is critical. It is a testimonial to the passion of the young scientists that come to my lab who are so driven by the enormous potential of ES cells that they are willing to work diligently despite the uncertainties intrinsic to the current policy. It is the spirit of scientific passion and enthusiasm, combined with a truly generous financial commitment to health care research by our Federal Government that has made American science and our health care system the envy of the world. As a Nation, we should not miss the opportunity to nurture and invigorate this exciting field of medical research.

Thank you.

[The statement follows:]

PREPARED STATEMENT OF DR. GEORGE Q. DALEY

Distinguished members of the subcommittee. Thank you for the opportunity to address you this morning.

My name is George Daley. I am an Assistant Professor of Medicine at Harvard Medical School, a Research Fellow at the MIT-affiliated Whitehead Institute, and a staff hematologist at the Massachusetts General Hospital and the Children's Hospital in Boston. I run a research laboratory that studies stem cells that the body uses to form blood. We aim to understand how blood stem cells become deranged in diseases such as leukemia as well as to understand how normal blood cells develop within the embryo. This has prompted our intense interest in using human embryonic stem cells—ES cells—in our research.

My laboratory has spent the last seven years using mouse ES cells to investigate how blood cells develop in the Petri dish. Recently our group has taken a step forward. We successfully transplanted mice with blood stem cells derived entirely from mouse ES cells. Then, in collaboration with my colleague Rudolf Jaenisch, we performed an important first demonstration of therapeutic cloning to treat a mouse with a genetic immune deficiency similar to the Bubble-boy disease. Our team plucked a cell from the tail of an afflicted mouse, used nuclear transfer to generate an ES cell line, used gene therapy to correct the genetic defect, and then performed blood stem cell transplants into disease mice. The repaired ES cells provided a source of immune cells and antibodies in the treated mice. Encouraged by this first proof-of-principle in mice, my team is eager to apply the same strategies to human ES cells. Our hope is that one day the process will be efficient, safe, and effective for treating patients with a variety of genetic and malignant bone marrow diseases.

However, over the past year the progress of my own team and of that of the research community has been palpably slowed, in part because of the frustrating lack of access to human ES cells, and in part due to the restrictive nature of the President's funding policy as mandated in his address of August 9, 2001.

I will make three points. First, the biomedical research community needs more cell lines. While the President announced that over 60-odd cell lines were available as of August 9, 2001, it has become increasingly clear that far fewer lines have been characterized adequately. Some two thirds of the cell lines are located outside of the United States, and most are controlled by commercial entities. Currently, only a handful of lines are available to U.S. scientists.

Second, the biomedical research community needs a central repository for embryonic stem cell lines, preferably in a facility funded by NIH, that would serve the needs of the research community as a whole, providing free access to a comprehensive set of carefully maintained and documented human ES lines for research.

And third, I wish to emphasize that the federal funding guidelines are currently so restrictive that they are already threatening this fledgling yet highly promising field of biomedical research.

First, my personal experience. My team was one of the first in the United States to gain access to the human ES cells that Jamie Thomson and his colleagues derived at the University of Wisconsin. However, since obtaining a single line of cells in mid-2000, we have been frustrated in attempts to obtain additional lines. Many experiments require comparing the behavior of several different embryonic stem cell lines, since the behavior of any single line may be atypical and therefore highly misleading. One week ago, after nearly two years of inquiries with number of other research groups, we finally received a second cell line.

Why did it take so long? What are the hurdles that hinder sharing of these critically important research tools? What might be done to remedy the situation? The issues are complex. It is human nature that some scientists might wish to preserve their monopoly over these valuable cell lines. However, an accepted norm within our field, and a stipulation for publishing in most if not all journals, is that all research reagents will be made readily available to the research community to enable research results to be replicated and extended. Typically, when we request a research tool from a colleague in the research community, we receive it immediately, especially in this era of email and FEDEX. For all but a small handful of human ES cell lines listed on the NIH registry, this simply is not happening.

There is the perception that human ES cells hold significant commercial value given their potential for yielding products. Companies control most of the lines, and they have worked aggressively to dominate the intellectual property that flows from these cells. Thus, protracted negotiations over Material Transfer Agreements—called MTAs—have slowed the sharing of these lines with the wider research community. One of the most valuable initiatives performed by the U.S. Public Health Service and the NIH since August 9, 2001, was to negotiate with the University of Wisconsin a Memorandum of Understanding that provides a common set of terms for all federally funded researchers.

We have spent significant effort over the last two years negotiating MTAs with four different groups. Our most recent experience is a testimonial on how these negotiations should and can work. One of my post-doctoral scientists met Dr. Meri Firpo of the University of California, San Francisco, at a scientific meeting in August. Dr. Firpo had received a grant from the NIH to build an infrastructure to disseminate the lines, and graciously agreed to expedite our request. Our MTA negotiations were simplified by the prior agreements that had been hammered out by the NIH. Exactly 8 days ago, only some 6 weeks after originally speaking with Dr. Firpo, we received a second strain of human embryonic stem cells. We also received a handbook of detailed recipes for growing and maintaining the cells, and data on the characterization of the cell line. Clearly, Dr. Firpo is providing an exceptional service and her behavior should become a standard for how valuable embryonic stem cell lines are distributed to the scientific community.

The number of laboratories interested in working with these lines is already large and is increasingly explosively. This dictates that a more effective means must be established for the distribution of these valuable research reagents. I believe that a central warehouse and processing laboratory should be established and funded by the NIH to facilitate greater access to human ES cell lines for the general community of biomedical researchers. A central repository would maintain consistent standard operating procedures for the culture and maintenance of the cell lines. Strict quality control parameters would be established, and cell lines would be faithfully characterized under a uniform set of conditions. The Medical Research Council of the UK has just announced that it would fund such an effort in that country.

Finally, I wish to comment on the state of research on human ES cells after a year under the policy announced by President Bush last August 9, 2001. I would applaud President Bush for his principled stance in favor of human ES cell research. Having access to even a few well-characterized human ES cell lines enables many of us in the research community to begin to address generic questions about ES cell biology. We can make advances in cultivation of the cells, in coaxing the cells to become blood cells, neurons, insulin-producing cells, and the like. But this work is only the beginning, and the current policy will not enable the research community to follow-through with the work needed to treat patients. President Bush made the right call in allowing Federal funding for research, but his policy excludes some of the most important and promising avenues, and critical features of the policy are tying the hands of the research community.

First, the President announced that research support would be tendered only for cell lines that pre-existed before August 9, 2001. As I have stated, it is unclear precisely how many cell lines exist but I strongly believe that the number is far fewer than listed on the NIH registry. The President's policy prevents U.S. scientists from exploiting new cell lines as they become available. Scientists are by their very nature innovators, and hungry for the latest, most up-to-date technology and tools. All human ES cells listed on the NIH registry were derived in contact with mouse feeder cells. Scientists throughout the world are actively seeking to develop new cell lines that avoid this contamination, and would therefore be more valuable for generating human therapies. Indeed, scientists from Singapore have published the derivation of lines free of mouse cell contamination, but under the current policy, U.S. scientists can not study these cells using federal funds.

Second, the President's policy does not allow support for deriving new cell lines, which is of tremendous scientific interest. This is in stark contrast to the United Kingdom, whose scientists have made many of the seminal discoveries in ES cell biology and given their greater freedom are poised to dominate further. Our research community, hobbled by current restrictions, is falling behind researchers in other countries that are racing ahead to take full advantage of the possibilities that embryonic stem cells offer.

Third, the President's policy does not allow for studies of ES cell lines derived by nuclear transfer. This is currently the most appealing avenue for creating ES cells from patients with specific diseases, and for creating ES cell lines that are genetically matched to patients, which would overcome immune rejection of transplanted ES cell products. Our research team showed that nuclear transfer methods can be applied in the practice of therapeutic cloning in mice. I have no doubt that legitimate and successful medical treatments in real patients will be developed sooner if the Federal government funded nuclear transfer studies with human cells today. The sad and undeniable truth is that the existing restrictions are keeping these advances from being realized.

I realize that funding for some of these initiatives is currently prohibited by federal statute and that a change in legislation to specifically allow this work is needed. I applaud you Senator Specter, in your efforts to propose such legislation.

In conclusion, I would say that the field of human ES cell research is in a fragile state at best under the current Presidential policy. The current policy represents a half-hearted effort, and threatens to starve the field at a time when greater nourishment is critical. The scientists who come to train in my lab voice concerns that they might face inadequate research support in the future. It is a testimonial to the passion of these young scientists, who are so driven by the enormous potential of ES cells that they are willing to work diligently despite the uncertainties inherent under the current policy. It is that spirit of scientific passion and enthusiasm—combined with a truly generous financial commitment to health care research by our Federal government, that has made American biomedical science and our health care system the envy of the world.

Here at the beginning of the 21st century, we stand at the threshold of a new era in biomedicine, when cells will be harnessed to treat a wide array of degenerative conditions in an aging society. As a nation, we should not miss the opportunity to nurture and invigorate this exciting field of biomedical research.

Thank you for your time and interest in this matter.

Senator SPECTER. Thank you very much, Dr. Daley.

Dr. Zerhouni, we start with you on the questioning. You heard the testimony about the sharp limitations on the availability of stem cell research lines. In the fall of last year when NIH assembled the stem cell registry, it listed 78 stem cell lines from 14 sources around the world. According to the information which our subcommittee has been able to glean, only five of these lines are available to stem cell researchers. NIH has awarded, as you testified, $4.3 million in infrastructure grants to five companies and institutions with 23 eligible stem cell lines. Of these five companies, we are told only four have signed material transfer agreements with NIH, and these four companies have only 17 eligible stem cell lines. Of these 17 stem cell lines, only 5 have been shipped and are available to researchers.

Would you start the clock? We are going to have 5-minute rounds.

The question is, is there a sufficient number of stem cell lines available for the required research?

Dr. ZERHOUNI. Well, in terms of the number of eligible lines which is, as you said, 78, and the number of lines available for wide distribution, we would agree that over the year there has been an increasing number of lines. Last spring there was one. This month there are five. As far as we can tell from talking to all the suppliers, there are 10. I went over in my opening statement the time line that it takes to go from an eligible line that is just derived to a widely available distributable line.

So I think that progress is being made and we are, as mentioned by some of the researchers, diligently working with as many sources as we can to make more lines available.

Senator SPECTER. You are working with the sources of the 78 lines which were approved by the President as of August 9.

Dr. ZERHOUNI. Correct.

Senator SPECTER. And the question is, is that adequate? I know you are bound by the administration's decision, but the Congress has the authority to legislate in the field. The President may veto it but we can override a veto by two-thirds. In the spring of 2000, when NIH funding was not available on all of the stem cell research, Senator Harkin, myself, and others started a move, and we had letters signed by 64 Senators disagreeing with the Federal policy on stem cells. I had personal commitments from 12 more who were unwilling to put it in writing, but assured me that they would support legislation in the field.

Then the President came out with his compromise position. In essence, on August 9, and immediately after that, there was a flurry of publicity as to whether those lines were adequate. And the indications were at that time that they were not.

After September 11, all of the oxygen has been sucked out of Washington on virtually every other subject until Iraq came along to take some precedence. And we have been waiting to see the developments and have deferred this hearing, but now we are going to be faced with a decision as to what to do next.

So it is a pretty blunt question as to whether the existing stem cell lines are adequate. You have heard your colleagues at the table. What do you think?

Dr. ZERHOUNI. My feeling is that we are at a very early stage. It is actually not knowable how many lines you will need to advance the field. In other comparable fields, very often researchers want to limit the number of well-characterized lines that are used for experimentation.

So I would say at this moment, I do not think we know the answer. We need to work and develop more researchers and more laboratories that are going to experiment with the lines that we want to make available to find that answer. I really do not know the answer.

Senator SPECTER. Well, Dr. Zerhouni, when will we know? Can you give me a time line as to when we will know?

Dr. ZERHOUNI. We will work as diligently as we can to make as many lines available to as many laboratories. There is no limit to the funding that we can direct to the laboratories that present good, solid research proposals.

Senator SPECTER. Dr. Pedersen, to what extent do you think your example will be followed by others, in leaving the United States to go to places like Great Britain where you can get funding on stem cell research?

Dr. PEDERSEN. I cannot answer that exactly, Senator, but we are working as diligently as possible to recruit them.

Senator SPECTER. Have you had any success?

Dr. PEDERSEN. How I would like to answer that is in part a response to your prior question, which is how many cell lines are available to do the necessary work and how many are needed. There are, I think, adequate numbers of existing cell lines to do a portion of the work, the portion that will be focused on in the United States with Federal funding, namely, the characterization of the steps needed to get useful, specialized cells. So the dozen or so that are currently available, actually available probably are sufficient to do that.

I think this number issue is a red herring, though, because to go into patient care, the existing lines are not really useful because they have all been grown with a combination of mouse cells which makes them unsuitable for transplantation. So the actual number of suitable lines for transplantation is zero in the current set, and new lines must be generated. So the clinical delivery very likely will take place elsewhere and people who are interested in participating in that part of it will probably have to do so elsewhere.

Senator SPECTER. So you are saying the number of stem cell lines for clinical delivery, transplantation is zero.

Dr. PEDERSEN. On the registry is zero. There is one line that was developed recently in Singapore.

Senator SPECTER. Well, that could hardly be characterized as an adequate number.

Dr. PEDERSEN. And so the development of such lines in the U.S. would require a change in policy.

Senator SPECTER. My red light is on, plus 39 seconds from your last answer.

Senator Hutchison.

OPENING STATEMENT OF SENATOR KAY BAILEY HUTCHISON

Senator HUTCHISON. Well, thank you, Mr. Chairman, for holding this hearing, and I thank all of you for coming.

I am very concerned about the real-life stories. I always am interested when policies are set, and I think the President's policy was meant to be one that would allow for real use of the lines that are available so that we could do the testing that is necessary. But then I hear your stories about trying to get lines and then India does not let them out, and then you try to get a line in another way from Wisconsin and, yes, it is coming, well, no it is not, well, yes, it is later. That does not seem to be working in the practical sense.

I have researchers at UT Southwestern who are very concerned about availability. They are now doing work with animal nerve and pancreatic stem cells. They want to further that study, and they are very concerned about access.

So I would just ask you this question. I think that Senator Specter asked the big question, what can we do to make it more practically available? I think all of us are concerned about that.

On top of that, though, I now have another concern, and that is I have some great research institutions, M.D. Anderson, Baylor, UT Southwestern, UT San Antonio, UT Galveston. They are really on the cutting edge of research. Now California has stepped forward I think in a way that could start luring some of our good scientists to California, and I would like to ask you this question, Dr. Zerhouni.

Now that California is looking at giving State help in this regard and so many of our institutions are public institutions that do get private help but also need government help, what can we do to keep everything balanced so that all of a sudden we do not see people migrating from Harvard and Johns Hopkins and all these other great research institutions, including mine, all to the west coast? I am not saying I do not wish the west coast well. I do, but I do not want to, all of a sudden, throw a big kink in the research world. So tell me how we can deal with that effectively.

Dr. ZERHOUNI. Well, clearly I think, in terms of Federal funding, we need to look at all the aspects of facilitation of the research, and that is what we are doing. We have established the Stem cell Task Force where we can get input from the scientific community from all States as to exactly how we can, in fact, enhance the ability of these institutions to do the research. As Dr. Pedersen said, we need to do the basic research before we can go to clinical research. It will take years, but we need to do that.

In terms of State support and private support, there is nothing in the current policy that prevents that from happening. In California, for example, the UCSF lines were developed in part with State help.

Senator HUTCHISON. I understand that, Dr. Zerhouni. I know it is possible, but the amount that is available from private and State funds is not comparable to what could be available from Federal funds. So you are now looking at a potential problem I think even though private funds can be used, but it does become complicated, especially if you are doing a project that has Federal funds and then you want to take the next step. You want to go to the stem cell part that would actually show results. Do you have to stop doing the federally funded research?

Dr. ZERHOUNI. Currently we allow researchers to do side-by-side federally funded research and non-federally funded research in parallel. There is no NIH policy that prevents that as long as appropriate accounting mechanisms are in place. So I think that can still be done.

Senator HUTCHISON. And it can be the same, exact project. So you are on a project and the next thing you want to do is test it with embryonic stem cells, and you have a federally funded project. Can you use embryonic stem cells under the present law or the President's policy to do that research?

Dr. ZERHOUNI. As long as there is strict accounting of what is used. The present policy is very clear. You cannot use Federal funds for non-eligible lines, and you have to have in place accounting mechanisms which are clearly spelled out in our policies to be able to do that, but it is doable.

Senator HUTCHISON. I would like to ask other members of the panel if they feel that that differentiation is enough to allow people to go forward.

Dr. CIVIN. Senator Hutchison, I was thinking of a slightly different analogy, in terms of California, when I read this in the news, and I was hoping that Maryland would do the same thing and that other States would follow Justice Brandeis' suggestion I believe, that the States should be the laboratories of democracy in this area of stem cell research and that we should experiment with different solutions. I happen to think that the solution from the State of California is outstanding and would like to see that be the example for our Federal solution that is followed by the entire Government because this is where the money that will make the rubber hit the road will happen.

Very little funding realistically will come from the States for very much research. It has to be Federal funding for it to work. Ultimately it has to be a coherent Federal policy so that we can collaborate across the country on our research. But I see instead California as an example of a laboratory for democracy here.

Senator HUTCHISON. Dr. Schatten.

Dr. SCHATTEN. Senator Hutchison, thank you so much for these probing questions. I think we need to acknowledge that Dr. Zerhouni and the entire NIH is doing absolutely everything within their power, but it is not within their power. I know from my own experiences that in order for us to work on eggs that have failed to be fertilized from an IVF clinic, we need absolutely everything to be privately funded, even million dollar microscopes that we might use for just 10 minutes.

Many university administrators are terrified that their full Federal funding could be withdrawn if one investigator enters into an area that might pose a risk because of a confusion in how funds are either mingled or not commingled. I think really it is at this level, as Senator Specter has mentioned, that we could benefit from a clear national policy.

Thank you.

Senator HUTCHISON. Thank you.

I have seen the difference that the doubling of the NIH budget has made in the area of research, particularly into diseases that are not prolific diseases but nevertheless need to have research into them. I know that the availability of Federal funding is making a huge difference in the knowledge base that we have in medical research into so many diseases that have been ignored in the past.

So I would just say that I think Dr. Schatten's point is very good. I think NIH is doing everything they can. I think they are moving forward in every possible way with the policies that we have, but I just want to see what more we can do and also determine if something works in practicality after it is set forward.

I even think the President meant to do that. I think he said we are going to try this. This is the best way to approach it, in a very careful way, and he wanted to be careful because he values life so much. So I know his intentions were right, but I also think he left it open for us to come back and say—not me, but you, the research community and you, Dr. Zerhouni—he is going to look to you for advice to say did it work. How can we continue progress in a way that also gives value to human life? I think we just have to keep working on input from the research community and creativity, which I think Senator Specter is showing in trying to create a bank at NIH perhaps with some of these lines to make sure that they do not get into legalistic delays and bureaucratic stumbling that stop progress in America.

I want this research to be done in America, and I want you to come home.

Senator SPECTER. Thank you very much, Senator Hutchison.

We are now about 9 minutes into a 15-minute vote, so we are going to have to adjourn, as I had mentioned earlier.

What I would like you to do, Dr. Schatten, Dr. Civin, Dr. Daley, Senator Ortiz, and Dr. Pedersen, is to provide in writing what you would like to have available. You, Dr. Daley, talked about nuclear transfer studies. I would like to get the specifics as to what you have in mind. Dr. Civin commented about waiting a year for lines and he has not gotten them yet. Dr. Schatten talked about not enough lines available and worried about therapeutic cloning, as Senator Ortiz said.

I believe that the legislation passed by the House imposing criminal penalties on nuclear transplantation, or so-called therapeutic cloning, will not come to pass. We have stopped it in the Senate. We may have 60 votes if there is time on the calendar to pass a bill which would permit nuclear transplantation.

I think Senator Hutchison summarized the matter well. The President took a significant step on August the 9 in permitting some Federal funding. He was subjected to a lot of criticism. It is pretty hard not to be criticized on virtually anything the President or any of us in elective office do, so we are used to that. But then we have to see what has happened.

I would like you to respond specifically to what you would like to see done. Senator Ortiz, you have special insights into legislation. Give me your insights as to what legislation you would like to see done.

My own sense at the moment is that Congress is going to have to legislate on the subject. We had waited for a year-plus to see the experience.

Dr. Zerhouni, if you can supplement what you have said with a time line as to when you think you might know, we would be interested to know that.

But I think the time has come to legislate in the field. As I said, last year we had 64 Senators in writing and commitments from 12 more, and 12 and 64 are 76, which is 9 more than 67. So we are in a position to move where the need is sufficiently great.

I think this testimony has been very, very helpful. I think we have gotten the kernel of it, and your written answers will give us the balance. So thank you all very much for coming in.

ADDITIONAL SUBMITTED STATEMENT

We have received the prepared statement of Senator Larry Craig which will be placed in the record.

[The statement follows:]

PREPARED STATEMENT OF SENATOR LARRY CRAIG

Mr. Chairman, I would like to thank you for holding this hearing today to spotlight stem cell research. I would also like to thank all of our witnesses here today for taking the opportunity to address this very complex issue.

Stem cell research continues to offer a great deal of promise. This research could lead to exponential improvements in the treatment of many terminal and debilitating conditions. In many cases, researchers are already beginning to see the promise of this research.

With the President's decision last year to allow federal funds to be used to support research on existing stem cell lines, researchers have begun to make progress. Many scientists in this field of research confirm that there are ample number of cell lines available to fully understand how these cells work. We must encourage more researchers to take advantage of this historic opportunity.

Researchers are in the early stages of this process. It is a difficult science and should be dealt with at an appropriate pace. Many will say that this process is moving too slowly. However, there are many scientific hurdles that will have to be surmounted before we get to the point of actually replacing damaged tissues in the body and understanding the potential for clinical applications. This could take years. But we should invest the time and resources into doing what it takes to get to that point.

I understand that NIH has made a good-faith effort to facilitate the use of the existing stem cell lines and has created a framework to enable researchers to begin stem cell research in the United States. Understanding that there are many obstacles that must be overcome before major strides are made, we must be as supportive of this research as possible.

Again, I thank the Chairman for holding this hearing and look forward to learning more about the developments in this important research.

CONCLUSION OF HEARING

Senator SPECTER. Thank you all very much for being here, that concludes our hearing.

[Whereup...
ing was con...
vene subject...